YOUR KNOWLEDGE HAS VALUE

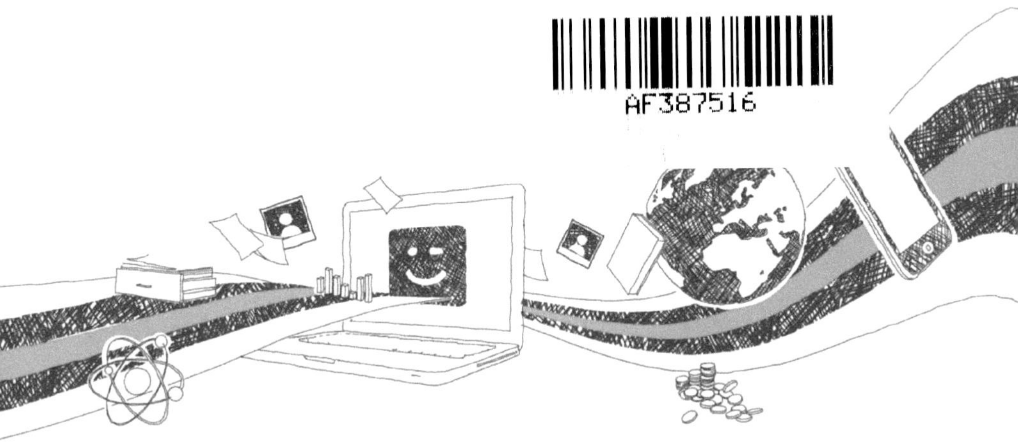

- We will publish your bachelor's and
  master's thesis, essays and papers

- Your own eBook and book -
  sold worldwide in all relevant shops

- Earn money with each sale

Upload your text at www.GRIN.com
and publish for free

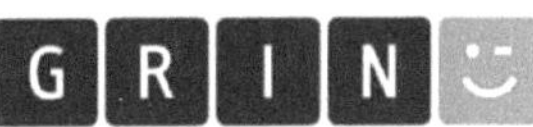

William Opoku-Nkoom

Case Study Report of Dietary Management of Severe Acute Malnutrition

GRIN Publishing

Bibliographic information published by the German National Library:

The German National Library lists this publication in the National Bibliography;
detailed bibliographic data are available on the Internet at http://dnb.dnb.de .

This book is copyright material and must not be copied, reproduced, transferred,
distributed, leased, licensed or publicly performed or used in any way except as
specifically permitted in writing by the publishers, as allowed under the terms and
conditions under which it was purchased or as strictly permitted by applicable
copyright law. Any unauthorized distribution or use of this text may be a direct
infringement of the author s and publisher s rights and those responsible may be
liable in law accordingly.

Imprint:

Copyright © 2010 GRIN Verlag GmbH
Print and binding: Books on Demand GmbH, Norderstedt Germany
ISBN: 978-3-656-84588-1

This book at GRIN:

http://www.grin.com/en/e-book/284147/case-study-report-of-dietary-management-
of-severe-acute-malnutrition

GRIN - Your knowledge has value

Since its foundation in 1998, GRIN has specialized in publishing academic texts by students, college teachers and other academics as e-book and printed book. The website www.grin.com is an ideal platform for presenting term papers, final papers, scientific essays, dissertations and specialist books.

Visit us on the internet:

http://www.grin.com/

http://www.facebook.com/grincom

http://www.twitter.com/grin_com

DIETARY MANAGEMENT OF SEVERE ACUTE MALNUTRITION: A CASE STUDY REPORT

WILLIAM OPOKU-NKOOM, MPHIL

NUTRITION AND FOOD SCIENCE DEPARTMENT, UNIVERSITY OF GHANA, LEGON

ABSTRACT

Severe acute malnutrition or severe wasting is defined as weight–for–length less than – 3 SD based on WHO standards. The condition is highly prevalent in populations living in the context of poverty with concurrent disease burdens. The worldwide prevalence of severe wasting in children below five years is estimated to be 35% and 2% in Ghana. Treatment of severe acute malnutrition is either facility– or hospital–based if there are complications and appetite is poor, or community–based in the absence of complications coupled with good appetite. In order to be abreast with the treatment of severe acute malnutrition, as part of the requirement in the masters program in nutrition at the University of Ghana, a marasmic case was identified at the Princess–Marie Louis Children's hospital in Accra-Ghana, and treatment monitored for two weeks. It was found that severely malnourished children have high risk of getting infections, as tuberculosis was diagnosed in the child by the second week. For success in the treatment of severe acute malnutrition, close medical attention is very imperative.

TABLE OF CONTENTS

Page

CHAPTER 1: INTRODUCTION ....- 3 -

CHAPTER 2: LITERATURE REVIEW ....- 4 -

2.1 DIAGNOSES OF SEVERE ACUTE MALNUTRITION ....- 4 -

2.2.1 DIAGNOSTIC TESTS...- 6 -

2.2.2 FORMULA DIETS FOR SEVERELY MALNOURISHED CHILDREN ....- 7 -

2.2.3 FEEDING THE SEVERELY MALNOURISHED ON ADMISSION ....- 8 -

2.2.4 DOS AND DON'TS IN THE MANAGEMENT OF SAM BASED ON WHO GUIDELINES ......- 9 -

2.2.5 NUTRITIONAL REHABILITATION ....- 10 -

CHAPTER 3: METHODOLOGY ....- 11 -

3.1. IDENTIFICATION OF CASE ....- 11 -

3.2. HISTORY AND SOCIO-DEMOGRAPHIC CHARACTERISTICS ....- 11 -

3.3. SCREENING/DIAGNOSTIC TESTS ....- 11 -

3.4. DIET OF THE CASE ....- 11 -

3.5. DIARY MEDICAL ROUTINE ....- 12 -

CHAPTER 4: RESULTS ....- 13 -

4.1. SOCIO-DEMOGRAPHIC CHARACTERISTICS..- 13 -

4.2. MEDICAL HISTORY ....- 13 -

4.3. DIETARY HISTORY ....- 14 -

4.4. DIETARY CHANGES AFTER ONSET OF ILLNESS AND ADMISSION ....- 14 -

4.5. PHYSICAL EXAMINATION ....- 15 -

4.6. DIAGNOSTIC TESTS...- 17 -

4.7. SPECIFIC TREATMENTS ....- 17 -

CHAPTER 5: DISCUSSION..- 18 -

5.1. DIET ON ADMISSION ....- 18 -

5.2. FAILURE TO RESPOND TO TREATMENT...- 19 -

5.3. HYPOTHERMIA ....- 20 -

5.4. LIMITATIONS OF THE STUDY ....- 21 -

CHAPTER 6: CONCLUSIONS AND RECOMMENDATIONS ....- 22 -

6.1. CONCLUSIONS ....- 22 -

6.2. RECOMMENDATIONS ....- 22 -

REFERENCES...- 23 -

APPENDIX ....- 24 -

CHAPTER 1: INTRODUCTION

Severe malnutrition is both a medical and a social disorder. The medical problems of the child result in part, from the social problems of the home where the child lives. Malnutrition is the end result of chronic nutritional and emotional deprivation, when care-givers out of ignorance, poverty or family problems, are unable to provide a child with adequate nutrition and care. Successful management of the severely malnourished child requires that both medical and social needs are satisfied (WHO, 1999). If the illness is viewed as being only a medical disorder, it is most likely the child will experience relapse when he or she is discharged. Severe acute malnutrition occurs in families that have limited access to nutritious food and are living in unhygienic conditions, which increase the risk of repeated infections; and also people living in the context of poverty.

In spite of important advances in prevention and treatment, malnutrition continues to be a worldwide problem. Internationally, 55 million children under the age of five are estimated to be wasted, of whom 19 million (35%) are severely wasted or severely malnourished (Bhutta *et al.*, 2008). In Ghana, according to the Demographic and Health Survey (GDHS, 2009), 9 % of children under five are wasted, with 2 % severely wasted. According to the GDHS (2009) wasting is highest among children age 6-8 months (29 %) and is lowest among children age 48-59 months (3 %). Wasting in Ghana is more common in the Upper West (14 %), Northern (13 %) and Central (12 %) regions (GDHS, 2009).

The case study was aimed at acquiring knowledge on the management or the treatment of severe acute malnutrition (SAM). Specific objectives included studying how a marasmic child is treated using diet, getting knowledge on physiological, physical and behavioral changes in the treatment of marasmus; studying the socio-demographic characteristics of a marasmic child; and getting information on how some diseases are interlinked with SAM.

CHAPTER 2: LITERATURE REVIEW

2.1 DIAGNOSES OF SEVERE ACUTE MALNUTRITION

The WHO and UNICEF recommend the use of a cut-off for weight-for height of below -3 standard deviations (SD) of the WHO standards to identify infants and children as having Severe Acute Malnutrition (SAM). According to the WHO/UNICEF (2009), this indicator is highly specific because statistical theory shows that in a well-nourished population; only 0.13% of children will have a weight-for-height less than -3 SD, giving a specificity of more than 99% for this cut-off.

The WHO standards for mid-upper arm circumference (MUAC)-for-age show that in a well-nourished population there are very few children aged 6 – 60 months with a MUAC less than 115 mm. Children with a MUAC less than 115 mm have a highly elevated risk of death compared to those who are above. Therefore the recommendation in using MUAC to define SAM is a cut-off point 115 mm. The prevalence of SAM based on weight-for-height below -3 SD of the WHO standards and those based on a MUAC cut-off of 115 mm, are very similar (WHO, 2009). This gives a high specificity of more than 99% over the age range of 6-60 months (WHO, 2009). These recommendations: weight-for-height z-score and MUAC-for-age are based on the new WHO child growth standard curves (WHO, 2006).

The presence of a bilateral pitting edema in children aged 6-60 months is also an independent indicator of SAM that requires urgent attention (WHO, 1999).

2.2 MANAGEMENT OF SEVERE ACUTE MALNUTRITION BY WHO GUIDELINES

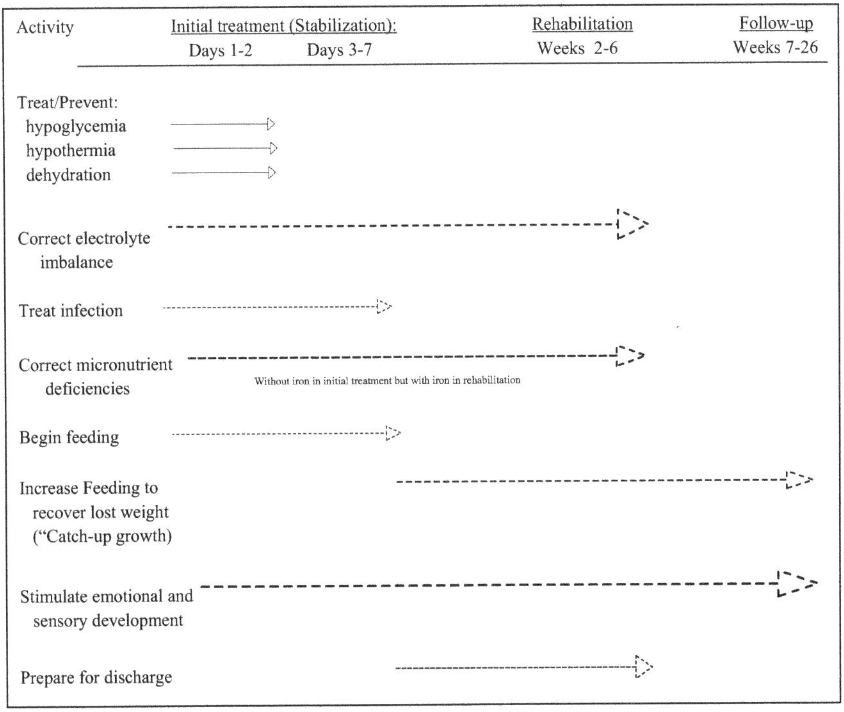

Activity	Initial treatment (Stabilization):		Rehabilitation	Follow-up
	Days 1-2	Days 3-7	Weeks 2-6	Weeks 7-26
Treat/Prevent:				
hypoglycemia	⟶			
hypothermia	⟶			
dehydration	⟶			
Correct electrolyte imbalance	⟶			
Treat infection	⟶			
Correct micronutrient deficiencies	Without iron in initial treatment but with iron in rehabilitation ⟶			
Begin feeding	⟶			
Increase Feeding to recover lost weight ("Catch-up growth)			⟶	
Stimulate emotional and sensory development	⟶			
Prepare for discharge			⟶	

Source: WHO (1999)

2.2.1 DIAGNOSTIC TESTS

Where resources are available, some specific tests may be carried out to help diagnose specific problems; they are however, not needed to guide or monitor treatment. According to the WHO (1999), tests that may be useful are what have been enumerated in Table 1.

Table 1: Some useful diagnostic tests

Test	Result and significance
Blood glucose	Glucose concentration <54 mg/dl (3 mmol/l) is indicative of hypoglycemia
Examination of blood smear by microscopy	Presence of malaria parasites is indicative of infection
Hemoglobin or packed-cell volume	Hemoglobin < 40g/l or packed-cell volume < 12% is indicative of very severe anemia
Examination and culture of urine specimen	Presence of bacteria on microscopy (or >10 leukocytes per high-power field) is indicative of infection
Examination of feces by microscopy	Presence of *Giardia* cysts or trophozoites is indicative of infection
Chest X-ray	Pneumonia causes less shadowing of the lungs in malnourished children than in well-nourished children Vascular engorgement is indicative of heart failure. Bones may show rickets or fractures of the ribs
Skin test for tuberculosis	Often negative in children with tuberculosis or those previously vaccinated with BCG vaccine.
Serum proteins	Not useful in management, but may guide prognosis
Test for human immunodeficiency virus (HIV)	Should not be done routinely; if done, should be accompanied by counseling of the child's parents and result kept confidential
Electrolytes	Rarely helpful and may lead to inappropriate therapy

Source: WHO (1999)

2.2.2 FORMULA DIETS FOR SEVERELY MALNOURISHED CHILDREN

Almost all severely malnourished children have infections, impaired liver and intestinal function, and problems related to imbalance of electrolytes when first admitted to hospital. Because of these problems, they are unable to tolerate the usual amounts of dietary protein, fat and sodium. Therefore these children are fed with a diet that is low in these nutrients, and high in carbohydrate. The daily nutrient requirements of severely malnourished children are enumerated in Table 2. Two formula diets, F-75 and F-100, are used for severely malnourished children. F-75 (75 kcal or 315 kJ/100 ml), is used during the initial phase of treatment, while F-100 (100 kcal or 420 kJ/100 ml) is used during the rehabilitation phase, after the appetite has returned.

Table 2: Daily nutrient requirements for severely malnourished children

Nutrient	Amount per kg of body weight
Water	120–140 ml
Energy	100 kcal (420 kJ)
Protein	1–2 g
Electrolytes:	
Sodium	1.0 mmol (23 mg)[a]
Potassium	4.0 mmol (160 mg)
Magnesium	0.6 mmol (10 mg)
Phosphorus	2.0 mmol (60 mg)
Calcium	2.0 mmol (80 mg)
Trace minerals:	
Zinc	30mmol (2.0mg)
Copper	4.5mmol (0.3mg)
Selenium	60 nmol (4.7mg)
Iodine	0.1 mmol (12mg)
Water-soluble vitamins:	
Thiamine (vitamin B1)	70 mg
Riboflavin (vitamin B2)	0.2 mg
Nicotinic acid	1 mg
Pyridoxine (vitamin B6)	70 mg
Cyanocobalamin (vitamin B12)	0.1 mg
Folic acid	0.1 mg
Ascorbic acid (vitamin C)	10 mg

Pantothenic acid (vitamin B5)	0.3 mg
Biotin	10 mg
Fat-soluble vitamins:	
Retinol (vitamin A)	0.15 mg
Calciferol (vitamin D)	3 mg
α-Tocopherol (vitamin E)	2.2 mg
Vitamin K	4 mg

[a] Value refers to the maximum recommended daily intake   Source: WHO (1999)

2.2.3 FEEDING THE SEVERELY MALNOURISHED ON ADMISSION

The WHO and UNICEF recommends F-75 diet to all children during the initial phase of treatment. The child is given at least 80 kcal or 336 kJ/kg, but not more than 100 kcal or 420 kJ/kg per day. If less than 80 kcal (or 336 kJ/kg) per day is given, the tissues will continue to be broken down and the child will deteriorate. If more than 100 kcal (or 420 kJ/kg) per day is given, the child may develop a serious metabolic imbalance. Table A1 (in the appendix) shows the amount of diet needed at each feed to achieve an intake of 100 kcal (or 420 kJ/kg) per day. For example, if a child weighing 7.0 kg is given the F-75 diet every 2 hours, each feed is 75 ml. In the initial phase of treatment, the volume of F-75 fed at 130 ml/kg per day is maintained, but the frequency of feeding is gradually decreased and the volume increased for each feed until the child is being fed 4-hourly (6 feeds per day).

2.2.4 DOS AND DON'TS IN THE MANAGEMENT OF SAM BASED ON WHO GUIDELINES

Children with severe malnutrition are often seriously ill when they first present for treatment. Wasting, anorexia and infections are common. Successful initial management requires frequent, careful clinical evaluation and anticipation of common problems so they can be prevented, or recognized and treated at an early stage.

Recently admitted children are kept in a special area where they can be constantly monitored. Because they are very susceptible to infection, they are, if possible, isolated from other patients. The child is not kept near a window and windows are often closed at night. The child is often well covered with clothes, including a hat, and blankets. Washing is kept to a minimum and, if necessary, done during the day. When the child is washed he or she is dried immediately and kept at a room temperature of 25–30 °C (77–86 °F). This might seem uncomfortably warm for active, fully clothed staff, but is necessary for small, immobile children who easily become hypothermic. The principal tasks during initial treatment are:

- to treat or prevent hypoglycemia and hypothermia

- to treat or prevent dehydration and restore electrolyte balance

- to treat incipient or developed septic shock, if present

- to start to feed the child

- to treat infection

- to identify and treat any other problems, including vitamin deficiency, severe anemia and heart failure.

2.2.5 NUTRITIONAL REHABILITATION

The child is deemed to have entered the rehabilitation phase when his or her appetite has been restored. The principal tasks during the rehabilitation phase include:

- encouraging the child to eat as much as possible

- re-initiating and/or encouraging breastfeeding as necessary

- stimulating emotional and physical development; and

- preparing the mother or the care-taker to continue to take care of the child after discharge.

Criteria for transfer to a nutritional rehabilitation center include:

- eating well

- improved mental state: smiles, responds to stimuli, interested in surroundings

- sits, crawls, stands or walks (depending on age)

- normal temperature (36.5–37.5 °C)

- no vomiting or diarrhea

- no edema

- gaining weight: >5 g/kg of body weight per day for 3 successive days

    By the guidelines of WHO and UNICEF (2009), a malnourished child under treatment qualifies for transfer into a rehabilitation center if the child has good appetite, no medical complications and has attained at least 15-20% of the weight on admission.

CHAPTER 3: METHODOLOGY

3.1. IDENTIFICATION OF CASE

Following the recommendations of the WHO and UNICEF, a child was diagnosed of marasmus: weight-for-length = -4SD and admitted at the Princess-Marie Louise (PML) Children's Hospital in Accra, Ghana on 23rd March 2010. This patient was used for the case study.

3.2. HISTORY AND SOCIO-DEMOGRAPHIC CHARACTERISTICS

Information on socio-demographic characteristics; medical history, including immunization history; and dietary history, including breastfeeding practices; of the child were obtained by interviewing the mother, who was also the care-giver. Physical examination was also conducted.

3.3. SCREENING/DIAGNOSTIC TESTS

Some of the screening/diagnostic tests that were performed in accordance to the guidelines of the WHO were hemoglobin test for anemia, skin test for tuberculosis, and HIV test (both mother and child).These information were obtained from medical practitioner report at post.

3.4. DIET OF THE CASE

In accordance with the current recommendations of the WHO, the child was put on F-75 formula feeding, taken into consideration the weight of the child. Changes in diet since current illness began, were studied through information obtained from both the mother, and the Resident Dietician.

3.5. DIARY MEDICAL ROUTINE

Body temperature was routinely measured every 24 hrs at 6:00 am, 10:00 am, 2:00 pm, 6:00 pm, 10:00 pm and 2:00 am. Total food intake, taken into consideration total amount consumed minus amount vomited was recorded each day. The child was first subjected to 3-hourly feeding; the child was being fed at 8:00 am, 11:00 am, 2:00 pm, 5:00 pm, 8:00 pm, 11:00 pm, 2:00 am, and 5:00 am. After 3 days on admission, the child's feeding was changed to 4-hourly feeding: 8:00 am, 12:00 pm, 4:00 pm, 8:00 pm, 12:00 am, and 4:00 am. Total amount of food consumed at each feeding period was recorded and the overall amount calculated for every 24 hours.

CHAPTER 4: RESULTS

4.1. SOCIO-DEMOGRAPHIC CHARACTERISTICS

The case was a marasmic male child of 15 months old who was diagnosed of tuberculosis in the second week after admission. The parents of the child were Christians and stay in Damfa near Madina, a suburb of Accra. The child was admitted on 23rd March 2010 at the Princess-Marie Louis Children's Hospital in Accra, Ghana.

The father and the mother were respectively 55 and 48 years old. The father was a driver whiles the mother, both a trader and a farmer. The mother had had 14 pregnancies of which two were unsuccessful. At the time of interview she was using injectables as a birth control method. It was the mother who was the care-giver at the time of interview. Her highest level of education was primary school; she could neither read nor write.

Monthly family income was about GH¢100.00 at the time of interview. The mother cultivated crops such as cassava, maize, pepper, tomatoes, etc. She lived in a compound house containing five rooms. There were exactly 10 adults living in the same house. The house had a hand-dug well on which the inhabitants relied for their water supply. The house did not have any sanitation facility, so the inhabitants used the public KVIP in the town. There was no electricity in that house. The family of the case could not boast of any household amenities.

4.2. MEDICAL HISTORY

The child was known to have had umbilical cord bleeding since birth i.e. for one year. Report of severe anemia was also noted with mild diarrhea and vomiting even though this did not raise any alarm for additional medical attention. The child had never been able to sit on his own. He was immunized against tuberculosis at birth. At ages 6 weeks, 10 weeks and 14 weeks, he was also immunized against poliomyelitis. In addition, he also received vaccination against diphtheria/pertussis/hepatitis B first at 6 weeks of age, 10 weeks and 14 weeks after birth.

4.3. DIETARY HISTORY

The child had been exclusively breastfed for 1 year because he did not have any appetite for complementary feeding. Complementary feeding started few weeks (about 7 weeks) after 1 year. He often consumed cereal-based products like porridge often 30 ml per feed. Other foods included mashed yam, mashed cocoyam what is locally referred to as "*mpotompoto*", in addition to fish. For these kinds of foods, the child was consuming 1 slice of yam (about 5 g) per feed. Fruits like water melon were also being fed to the child.

4.4. DIETARY CHANGES AFTER ONSET OF ILLNESS AND ADMISSION

On his admission, the child was being fed on F-75. With F-75, the child was being fed 3-hourly and therefore received 8 feeds per day, 55 ml per feed and 440 ml per day. Eight-time feeding protocol begun from the day of admission to the 3rd day. He was being fed at 8:00 am, 11:00 am, 2:00 pm, 5:00 pm, 8:00 pm, 11:00 pm, 2:00 am and 5:00 am. From the 4th day, the child was switched on to a 4-hourly feeding protocol, with an attained weight of 4 kg. This feeding protocol comprised a total consumption of 90 ml per feed, 540 ml per day. For this he was being fed at 8 am, 12 pm, 4 pm, 8 pm, 12 am and 4 am. The shift from 3-hour to 4-hourly feeding was because of no vomiting, little diarrhea and the fact that he finished all foods fed to him. This dietary regimen was consistent with WHO/UNICEF (2009) guidelines.

The child had a very good appetite and therefore was consuming all the food he was being fed. This formula feeding was also coupled with breastfeeding.

The child weighed 3.5 kg on admission and had a length of 62.5 cm. He had no edema but severely wasted with weight-for-length z score of -4 SD; and mid-upper-arm circumference of 79 mm. The hair appeared sparse and the skin looked wrinkled. He had low pulse and seemed to gasp for breath sometimes. The appearance of his feces was normal.

The weight of the child from admission to the end of following the case is plotted in Fig.1 below. Changes in body temperature are also plotted in Fig. 2.

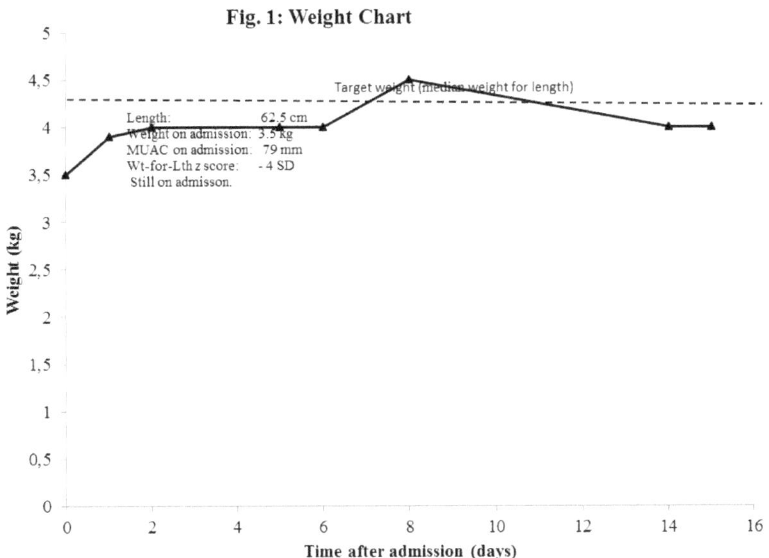

Fig. 1: Weight Chart

The child responded gradually by consistent increase in weight for exactly one week, after which he began to lose and maintain weight. He never seemed to be responding to treatment from that time forth and seemed far away from the target weight even after several days of stabilization.

Fig. 2: Temperature plot

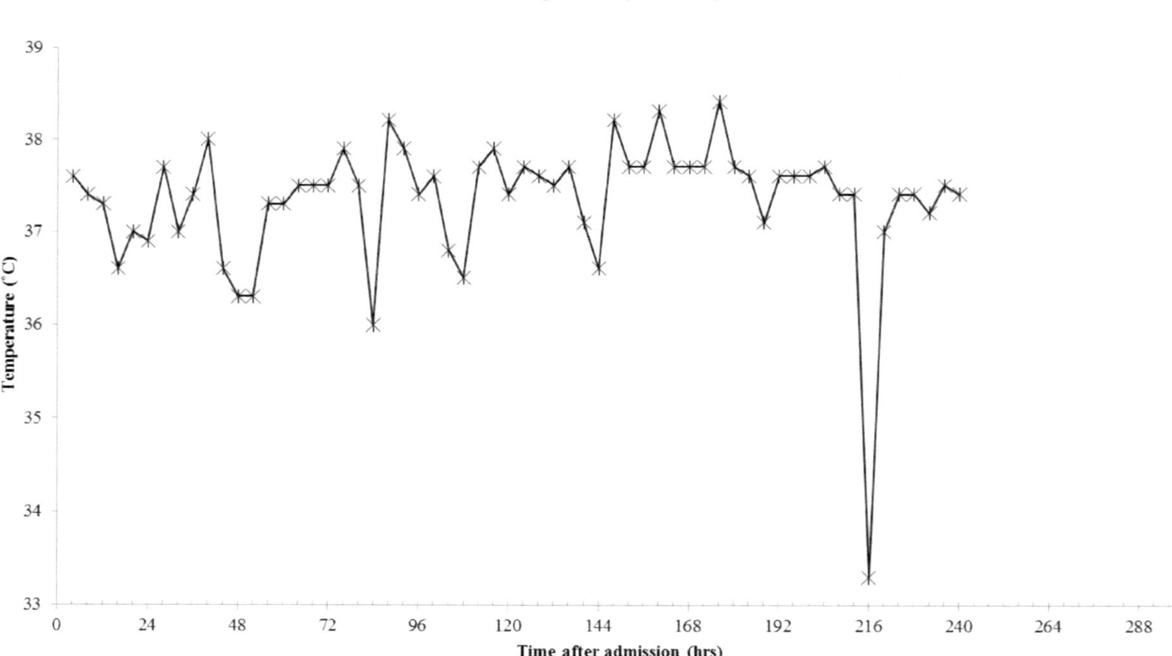

Body temperature was taken 6 times in a day at 6:00 am, 10:00 am, 2:00 pm, 6:00 pm, 10:00 pm and 2:00 am.

The child maintained normal body temperature most of the time but had occasional fever even though that was mild, on the 2nd, 4th and the 7th days after admission, but run into serious hypothermic state (temperature of 33.3°C against a normal temperature of 36.5-37.5) on the 9th day of admission.

4.6. DIAGNOSTIC TESTS

The child was diagnosed of severe anemia in the very early stages of treatment. Furthermore, he was diagnosed of tuberculosis on the 8th day of admission.

4.7. SPECIFIC TREATMENTS

The child was given blood transfusion for treatment of the severe anemia and also antibiotics like cloxacillin, gentamyacin, zincovate, and cefurosime for general infections which were not specified. For the tuberculosis the child was given antikocks for treatment.

CHAPTER 5: DISCUSSION

This was a marasmic case study at the Princess-Marie Louis Children's hospital in Accra, Ghana. For a child to be exclusively breast-fed for 12 months there was no wonder that this marasmic condition ensued. The current WHO recommendation on breastfeeding is exclusive breastfeeding for the first 6 months; and breastfeeding plus complementary feeding at 6 months and beyond. This is in recognition that from 6 months the breast milk alone is no longer adequate to support the high nutrient requirement of the growing child, and therefore cannot compensate for the growth spurt of children at this age. Good complementary foods are therefore required to provide the nutritional deficits of the breast milk. But as a result of an underlying disorder which was suspected to be congenital even though there were no records of this in the medical history, the child was denied of the necessary appetite for complementary feeding.

The socio-economic background of the parents might have also contributed to the marasmic condition. One's access to a medical facility is highly dependent on his or her socio-economic status. It was evident that the parents could not bear the cost of treatment of the bleeding umbilical cord and therefore could not access any appropriate medical facility for over a whole year. The situation might have also been worsened by the low educational background of the mother since this relates directly with the extent of wasting in under five children (GDHS, 2009).

5.1. DIET ON ADMISSION

The recommended feed for a severely malnourished admitted at the hospital is F-75, according to the guidelines of the WHO. This is normally used at initial or stabilization phase of the treatment. Throughout this case study, it is F-75 which was being given to the child. The nutrient composition of F-75 is consistent or meets the dietary nutrient requirement of the severely malnourished child (Table 2); it contains as part of the mineral composition sodium, potassium, magnesium, copper and zinc but no iron. There is potassium deficit in all malnourished children and this adversely affects cardiac functioning, and gastric emptying (WHO, 1999). Therefore, its presence in the diet is very important. The presence of magnesium in the diet is also very important since it is required for potassium to enter cells and be retained (WHO, 1999). The mineral composition of F-75 does not contain iron and is also not required as shown in Table 2. This is because severely malnourished children are highly susceptible to infections and iron is known to propagate microbial growth; therefore severely malnourished children are not given iron because of its toxic effects and reduced resistance to infections. It was very essential to feed the child frequently day and night; and in small quantities in order to avoid overloading the intestines, liver, and kidneys. This is because severely malnourished children have atrophied organs and overloading them may be fatal.

5.2. FAILURE TO RESPOND TO TREATMENT

As shown in Fig. 1, the child did not seem to be responding adequately to treatment especially after the 9th day of admission, after he had consistently shown some progress in his weight even though these changes were not drastic. According to Bhatnagar *et al.* (2007), poor weight gain is characterized by < 5 g/kg/day weight gain, and a good weight gain is characterized by >10 g/kg/day and indicates a good response. From Fig. 1 the child demonstrated good weight gain up to the 8th day after which he began to show poor weight gain. By the guidelines of the WHO reviewed by Bhatnagar *et al.* (2007), when a severely malnourished child begins to show poor weight gain, screening for inadequate feeding, untreated infection, tuberculosis and psychological problems are recommended. These recommendations were adhered to, and led to the diagnoses of tuberculosis in the second week of the treatment. Malnutrition is a major risk factor in the onset of active tuberculosis (Cegielski and McMurray, 2004). Research findings provide further support that malnutrition has an impact on the clinical outcome of tuberculosis (Singal *et al.*, 2005). Stimulation of an immune response by infection increases the demand for metabolically derived anabolic energy and associated substrates. This leads to adverse nutritional status due to energy loss in the individual (Schaible and Kaufmann, 2007). It was therefore evident that the growth failure was as a result of underlying tuberculosis infection.

There was tuberculosis infection despite an earlier vaccination against this disease. However, this observation is consistent with the results from animal study which found that the efficacy of BCG vaccination against tuberculosis was profoundly reduced in malnourished guinea pigs as compared to normally fed animals. This was largely attributed to impaired T cell priming and function in the context of malnutrition (McMurray *et al.*, 1999; Cegielski and McMurray, 2004).

5.3. HYPOTHERMIA

As shown in Fig. 2 for most times the child was within the normal temperature range of 36.5—37.5°C, however, on day 9 at 8:00 am, the child went into a serious hypothermic state (temperature of 33.4°C). It is not strange that the child went into this state of hypothermia, because all severely malnourished children are at elevated risk of hypothermia especially in the presence of concurrent infections and denuded skin, due to a lowered metabolic rate and decreased body fat (Bhatnagar *et al.*, 2006). Attention is drawn to the fact that it was around the same period that tuberculosis was diagnosed and lack of response to treatment was detected. Prevention of hypothermia in the treatment of severe malnutrition is therefore very crucial. However, in the presence of hypothermia it is recommended that hypoglycemia is screened and managed. There were however, no records of management of hypoglycemia in this case study.

5.4. LIMITATIONS OF THE STUDY

This study is limited by the fact that it was a short-term study and the patient was not monitored for a long time. Moreover, the whole study was restricted to the stabilization phase because of underlying tuberculosis infection which seemed to prolong the phase. Lack of time did not permit for continuous monitoring at the rehabilitation and the follow—up phases. That notwithstanding, the objectives of this case study were well achieved.

CHAPTER 6: CONCLUSIONS AND RECOMMENDATIONS

6.1. CONCLUSIONS

A great deal of caution is required in the treatment or the management of the severely malnourished child, in terms of dietary composition i.e. specific nutrients that are indispensable like potassium and magnesium and those that need to be excluded like iron. Care is also needed in the type of feed in terms of overall caloric contribution at the various stages of treatment, and the frequency of feeding. Close monitoring of variables such as temperature as a daily routine and some diagnostic tests or screening cannot be over emphasized for the successful treatment of the severely malnourished child.

This case study also supports the finding that independent of HIV, socioeconomic factors and tuberculosis, are important correlates of acute protein energy malnutrition or wasting (Villamor, *et al.*, 2006).

6.2. RECOMMENDATIONS

1. It is highly recommended that in the treatment of the severely malnourished, guidelines are adhered to strictly.

2. Efforts should be made in preventing easily avoidable complications like hypothermia.

3. Efforts should be made in preventing any further infections in the treatment of the severely malnourished.

REFERENCES

Bhatnagar, S., Lodha, R., Choudhury, P., Sachdev, H. P. S., Shah, N. S., Wadhwa, N. N., Makhija, P., Kunnekel, K. and Ugra, D. (2007). IAP Guidelines 2006 on Hospital Based Management of Severely Malnourished Children (Adapted from the WHO Guidelines). *Indian Pediatrics* 44:443—61.

Bhutta, Z. A., Ahmed, T., Black, R. E. (2008). What Works? Interventions for Maternal and Child Undernutrition and Survival. *Lancet*; 371:417–40.

Cegielski, J. P. and McMurray, D. N. (2004). The relationship between malnutrition and tuberculosis: Evidence from studies in humans and experimental animals. *Int J Tuberc Lung Dis* 8: 286–298.

Ghana Demographic and Health Survey (2009). 2008 edition. Nutrition of Children and Adults. Pp 179 183.

McMurray, D. N., Dai, G., and Phalen, S. (1999). Mechanisms of vaccine-induced resistance in a guinea pig model of pulmonary tuberculosis. *Tuber Lung Dis* 79: 261–266.

Schaible, U. E. and Kaufmann, S. H. E. (2007). Malnutrition and Infection: Complex Mechanisms and Global Impacts. *Plos Medicine* 4 (5) e 115.

Singal, A., Pandhi, D., and Agrawal, S. K. (2005). Multifocal scrofuloderma with disseminated tuberculosis in a severely malnourished child. *Pediatr Dermatol* 22: 440–443.

Villamor, E., Saathoff, E., Mugusi, F., Bosch, R. J., and Urassa, W. (2006) Wasting and body composition of adults with pulmonary tuberculosis in relation to HIV-1 coinfection, socioeconomic status, and severity of tuberculosis. *Eur J Clin Nutr* 60: 163–171.

WHO Multicentre Growth Reference Study Group (2006): WHO Child Growth Standards: Length/ height-for-age, weight-for-age, weight-for-length, weight-for-height and body mass index-for-age: Methods and development. Geneva, World Health Organization. Available at: http://www.who. Int/childgrowth/standards/technical_reporten/ index.html.

WHO/UNICEF (2009). WHO Child Growth Standards and the Identification of Severe Acute Malnutrition in Infants and Children: A joint statement by the WHO and the UNICEF.

World Health Organization (1999). Management of severe malnutrition: a manual for physicians and other senior health workers. Geneva. Available at: http://www.who.int/nutrition/ publications/en/manage_severe_malnutrition_ eng.pdf

Table A1: Determining the amount of diet to give at each feed to achieve a daily intake of 100 kcal or 420 kJ/kg

Weight of child (kg)	Volume of F-75 per feed (ml)[a]		
	Every 2 hours (12 feeds)	Every 3 hours (8 feeds)	Every 4 hours (6 feeds)
2.0	20	30	45
2.2	25	35	50
2.4	25	40	55
2.6	30	45	55
2.8	30	45	60
3.0	35	50	65
3.2	35	55	70
3.4	35	55	75
3.6	40	60	80
3.8	40	60	85
4.0	45	65	90
4.2	45	70	90
4.4	50	70	95
4.6	50	75	100
4.8	55	80	105
5.0	55	80	110
5.2	55	85	115
5.4	60	90	120
5.6	60	90	125
5.8	65	95	130
6.0	65	100	130
6.2	70	100	135
6.4	70	105	140
6.6	75	110	145
6.8	75	110	150
7.0	75	115	155
7.2	80	120	160
7.4	80	120	160
7.6	85	125	165
7.8	85	130	170
8.0	90	130	175
8.2	90	135	180
8.4	90	140	185
8.6	95	140	190
8.8	95	145	195
9.0	100	145	200
9.2	100	150	200
9.4	105	155	205
9.6	105	155	210
9.8	110	160	215
10.0	110	160	220

[a] Rounded to the nearest 5 ml.

Source: WHO (1999)